You R Ripped
Juicing

GREATEST JUICES FOR WEIGHT LOSS

2 PROFESSIONAL MODELS SHARE THEIR SECRETS

FAT-BURNING JUICES

You R Ripped Juicing

Written by Ana Molisteanu & Kristófer Anderson

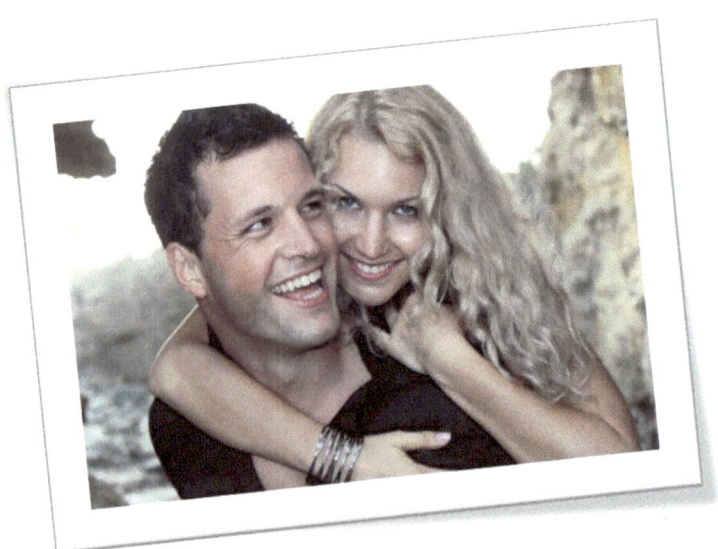

Juicing...

Cleanses
Detoxify
Nourishes
Regenerates
Rejuvenates

What is Juicing and why is it so Important?

1. Juicing is a way to get all of the nutrients of leafy greens, vegetables, and fruits; without having to digest all of the dietary fiber. By drinking a juice, you are essentially allowing your body to **absorb all the nutrients of greens and vegetables**, without spending anytime breaking it down in the digestive system.

2. Juicing is one of the easiest ways to **provide high level of nutrients to your body!**

3. Juicing provides vital nutrients, antioxidants, vitamins and minerals for your body to repair itself. It **strengthens your immune system** and the **cell's regenerate and grow.**

4. Juicing **gives your digestive system a break.**

5. Juicing helps **detoxify your body and eliminate the toxins**, fats, preservatives and chemicals that a diet of processed foods leaves in your body.

6. Juicing allows your body to **absorb high-quality nutrients**, which leads to **increased energy levels**.

7. Juicing is the perfect way to **consume more vegetables**. If you do not eat enough vegetables or you do not like to eat vegetables, than juicing is the best way to get what the body needs. You will like it eventually and you will soon crave it. It is what the body ordered!

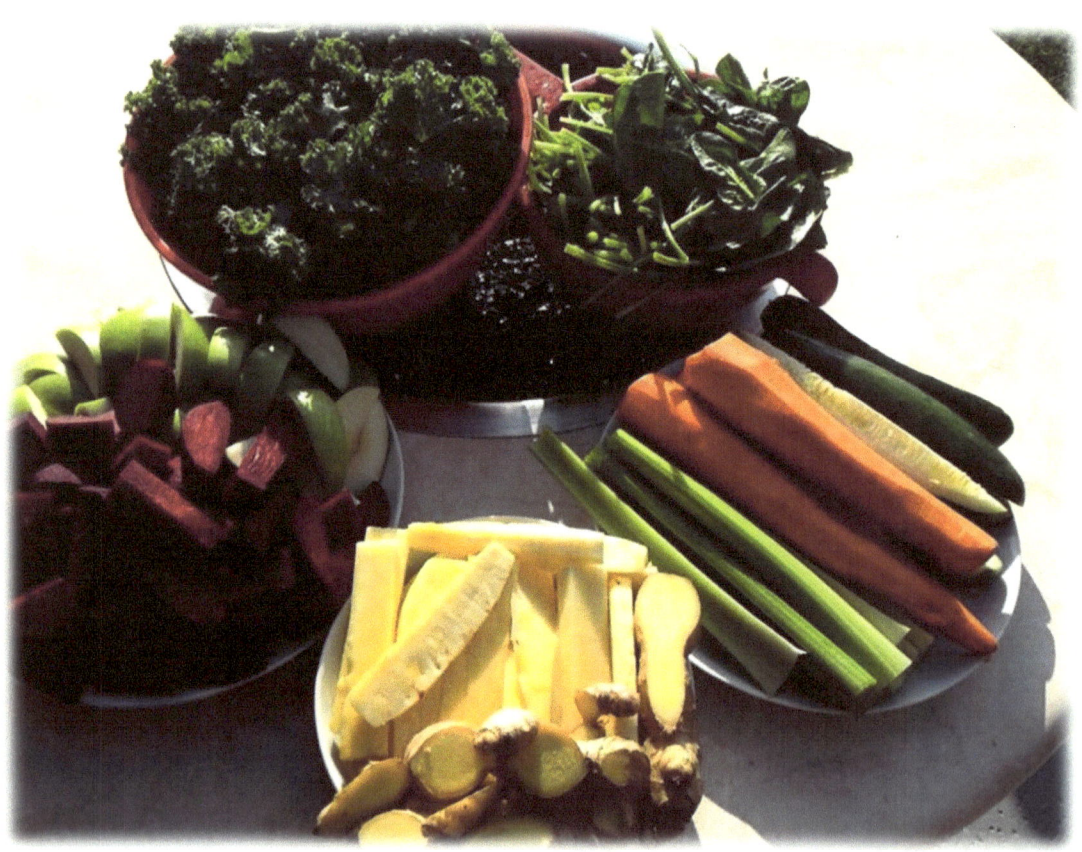

Chlorophyll in Greens
Blood Builder and Purifier!

Chlorophyll is a phytochemical that makes plants green. This green molecule is powerful and works like an internal healer, cleanser, antiseptic, cell stimulator, cell rejuvenator and red blood cell builder.

Researchers have reported that the chlorophyll molecule is remarkably similar to hemoglobin in human blood, the substance that carries oxygen in our body, which gives energy to the cells.

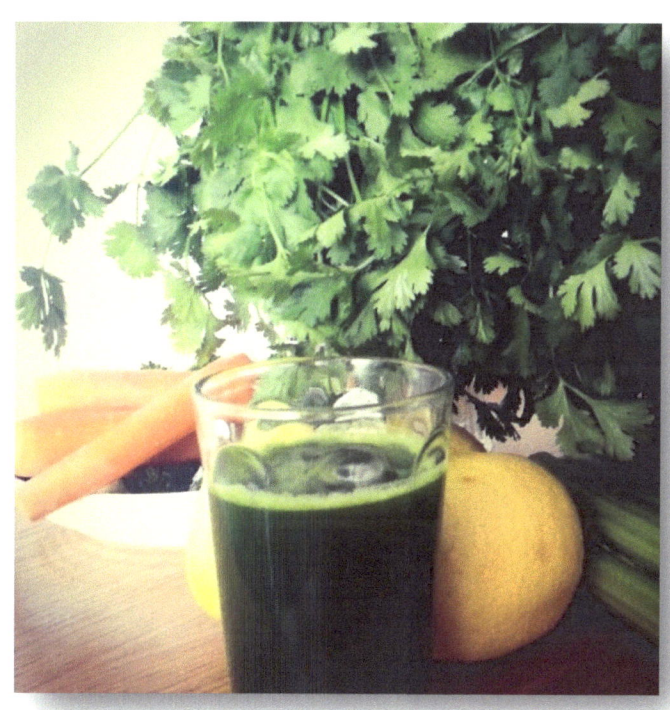

Chlorophyll has so many benefits. Some of them are:

- Detoxifies and cleanses
- Increases blood count
- Reduces or eliminates body odors
- Greatly relieves respiratory troubles
- Kills bacteria in wounds and speeds up healing
- Reduces inflammation pain
- Improves bowel functions
- Improves milk production in lactating mothers

More Juicing benefits...

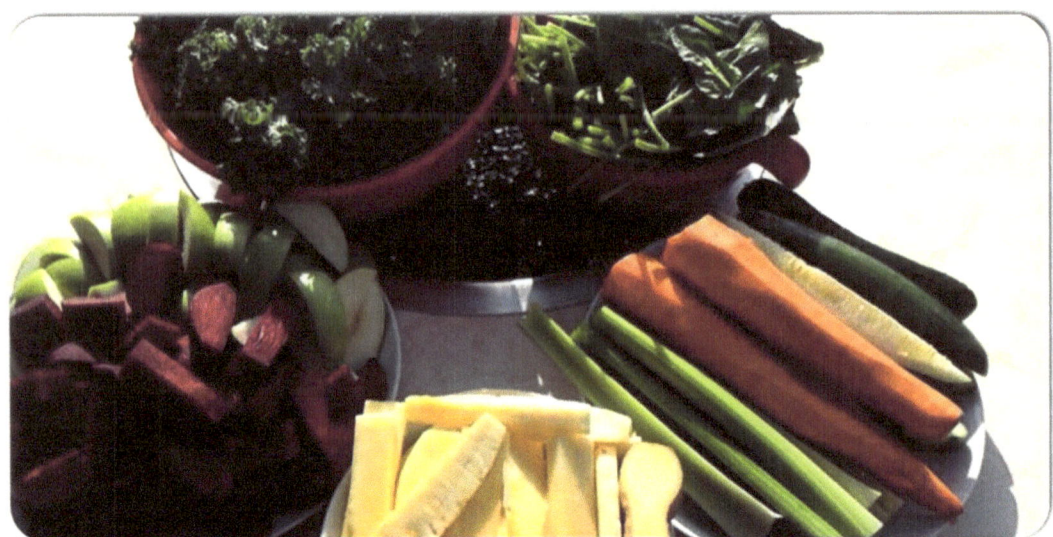

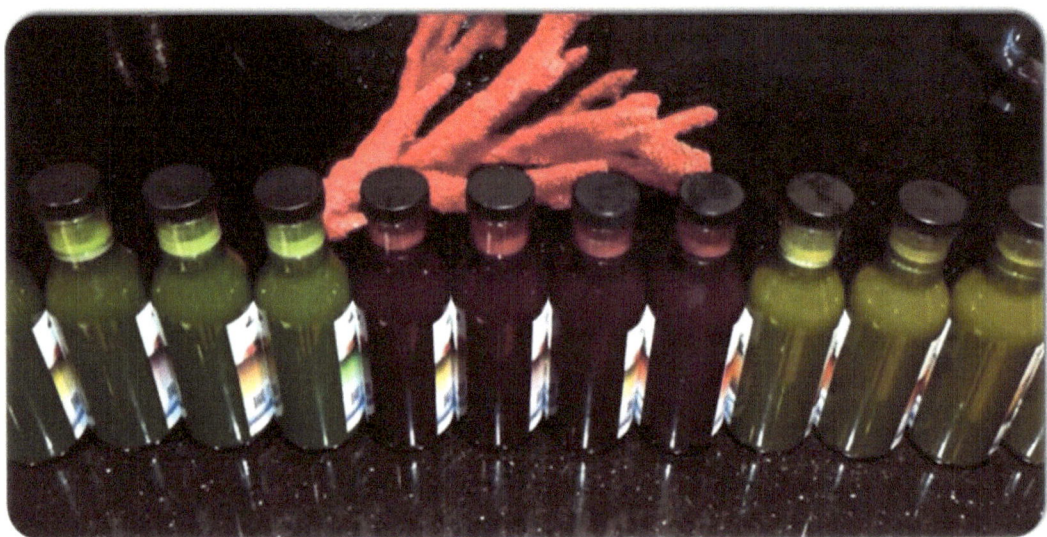

- Juicing makes you feel magically more vibrant, alive and energized.
- Consuming vegetables and fruits in the form of juices will definitely add years and years to your life!
- Juicing "connects the **BODY, MIND** and **SPIRIT**".
- Juicing awakens the HAPINESS from the inside and shows the BEAUTY on the outside!
- "Makes your life Juicy!"

JUICING DETOX
PROGRAM

The Detox cleanse can be a one day program, multiple day, week long or month long program. Speak with your local doctor before starting this or any detox and exercise program.

Start the day with 2 large cups of fresh drinking water! Squeeze a lemon or lime to add flavor. To kick up your metabolism, add a pinch of cayenne pepper!

Drink at least 6 Juices per day, one juice every 2-3 hours or when you feel hungry!

Remember to drink water throughout the day!

Take it easy and don't exercise too hard. Go for a walk, do some yoga or another stretching routine.

You can juice different ingredients to make your own juices according to your taste! Always use more vegetables than fruit!

Don't drink coffee, Don't smoke and Don't use any other stimulants During your detox program!

What can I expect from a Juicing Detox or Cleanse?

You might experience some withdrawals and cravings during the body detox process. Headaches are common in the initial stage. This is caused by all the toxins we ingest through processed foods, sugar, meats, smoking, wheat, dairy, and soy. This is normal.

The Good News

As soon as the benefits of the juices start to kick in, you will experience more energy, lose weight, and have clear skin. Your body will have a stronger immune system leaving you less susceptible to contracting illnesses. Your taste buds will improve and you will not have strong cravings for processed and sugary foods. Instead you will achieve healthier eating habits which will lead to a positive wellbeing and healthier lifestyle. You are going to feel great!

Juicing Preparation

Important tools for juicing: A good quality juicer, a strong knife, a peeler and a cutting board.

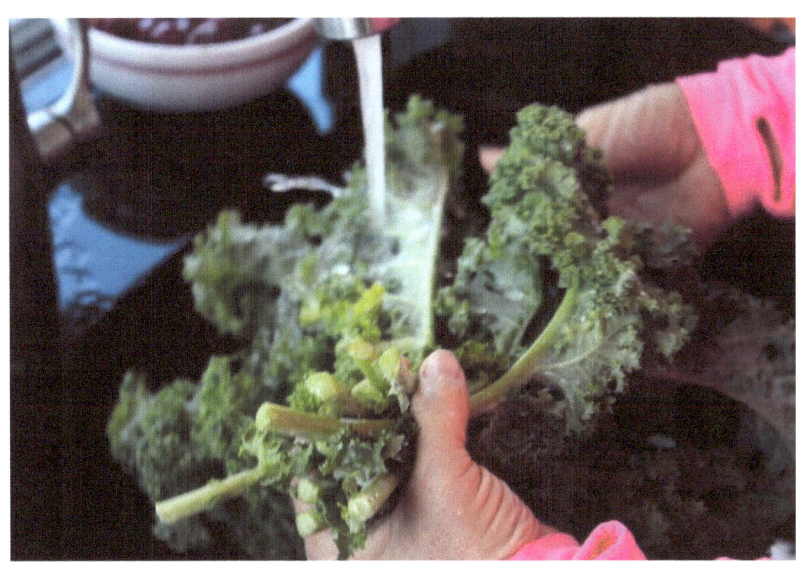

Step 1. Wash all the Ingredients well.

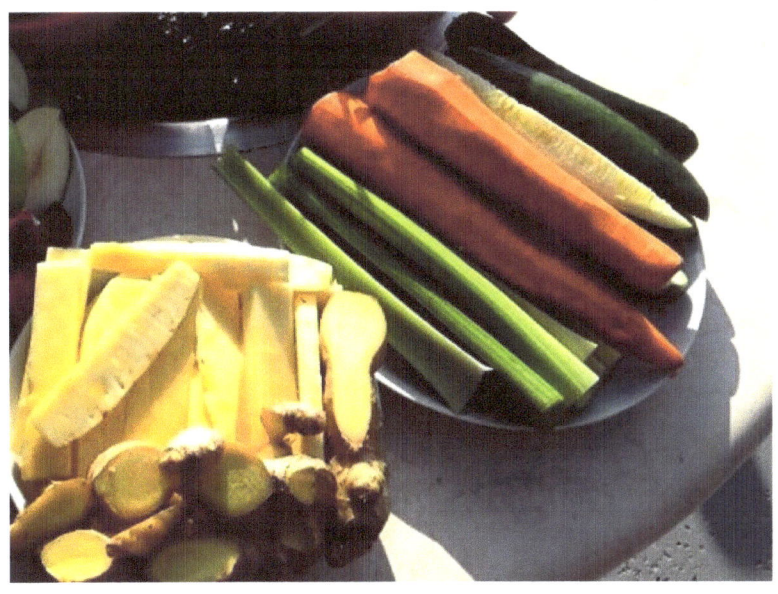

Step 2. Peel Carrots, oranges, grapefruit, lemons, etc...

Step 3. Cut ingredients into smaller pieces or slices, so they fit in the juicing machine.

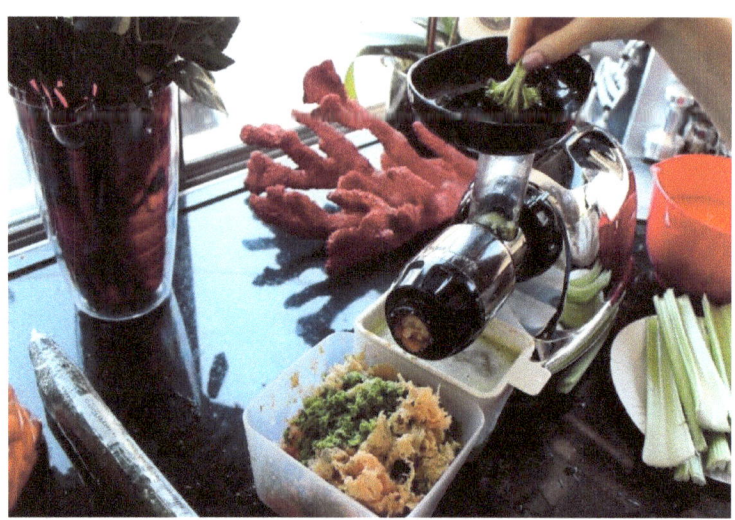

Step 4. Feed the fruits and veggies into the feeder.

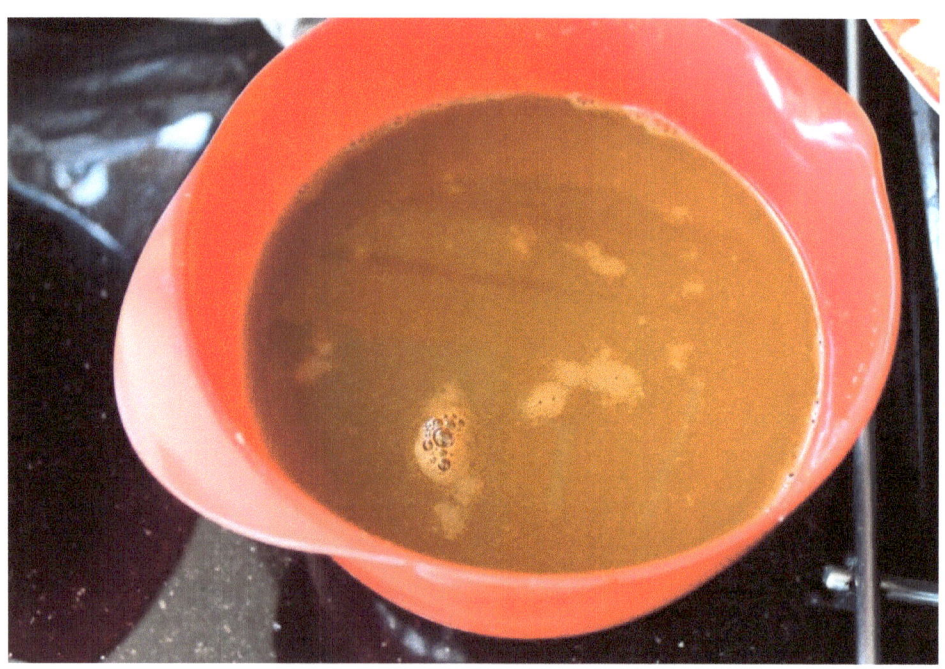

Step 5. Filter the juice and discard the excess.

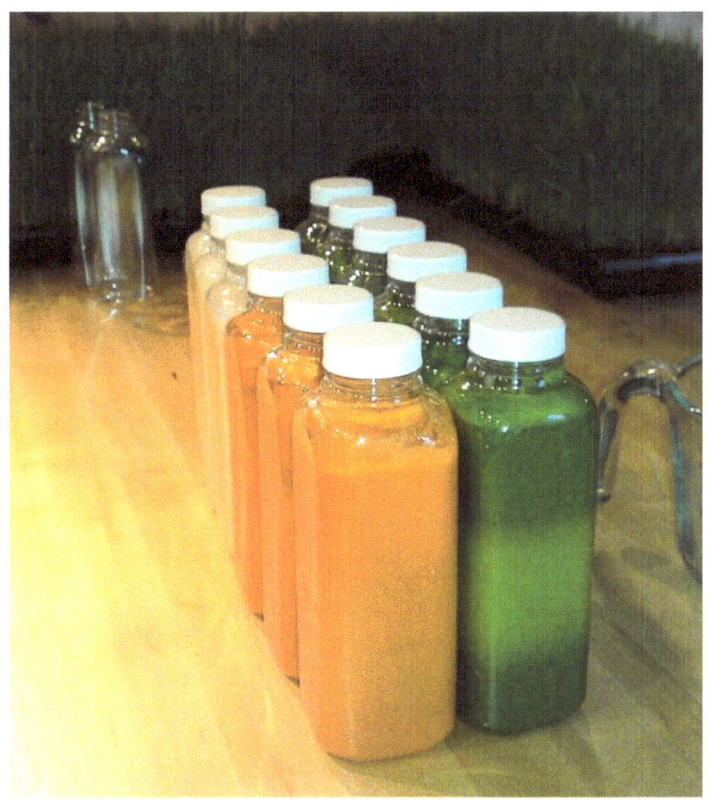

Step 6. Pour the juices in 16 oz. bottles and refrigerate. Juices will last 5 days, however it is best if consumed fresh at the time of juicing. You will absorb more nutrients this way.

Tip: You can also use the pulp from ingredients like carrots and apples to make healthy cookies or cakes. It is also safe to freeze the pulp if it's a big quantity.

Enjoy the finished juice!

Good Morning Drink

The Perfect drink to have as soon as you wake up.

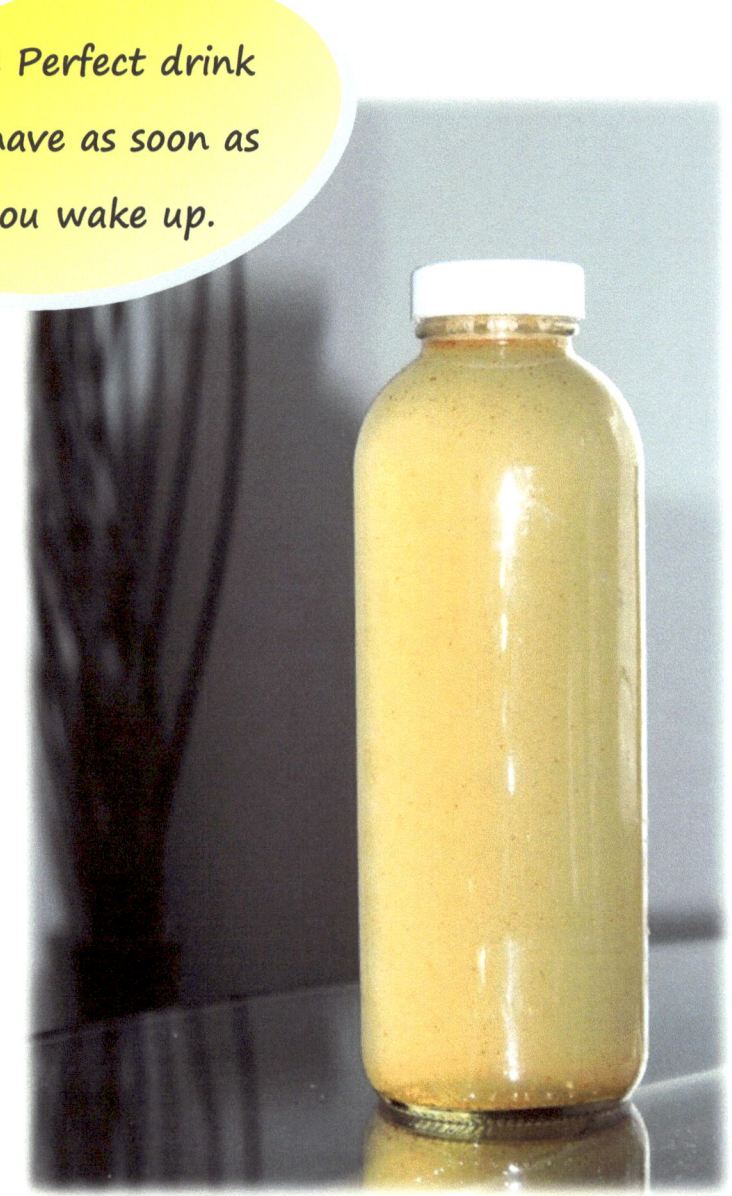

Ingredients:
- ✓ 12 oz. filtered water
- ✓ 2 tablespoons Maple Syrup
- ✓ 3 tablespoons Lemon Juice
- ✓ A dash of cayenne pepper (2 pinches)

Juice all the ingredients, mix together and enjoy!

Carrot Fuel

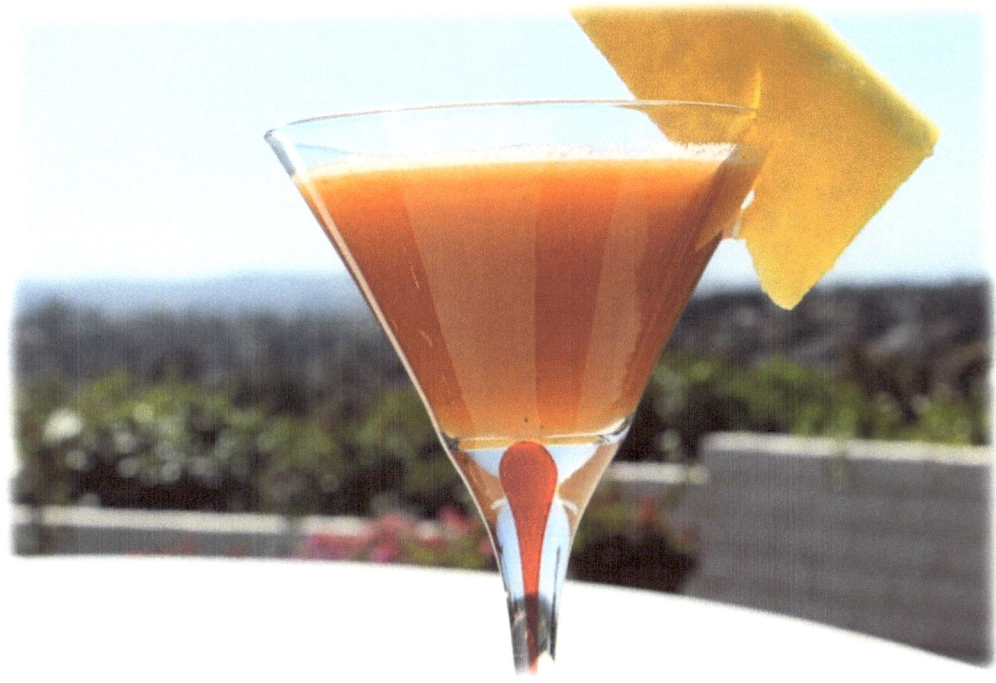

Ingredients:

- ✓ 9 Carrots (medium size)
- ✓ 2 Apples
- ✓ 1 Lime (peeled)
- ✓ 1 ½ inch Ginger piece

Directions:
Juice all the ingredients, mix together and enjoy!

Green Detox

Ingredients:

- ✓ 1 Cucumber
- ✓ 1 Bunch Kale Leaves
- ✓ 4 Stalks of Celery
- ✓ About 1/3 bunch Cilantro
- ✓ 1 ½ Limes (peeled)
- ✓ 4 cups Spinach
- ✓ 1 Apple

Directions:
Juice all the ingredients, mix together and enjoy!

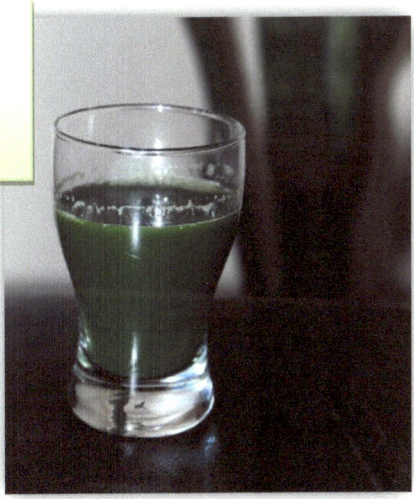

Apple & Carrot Pie

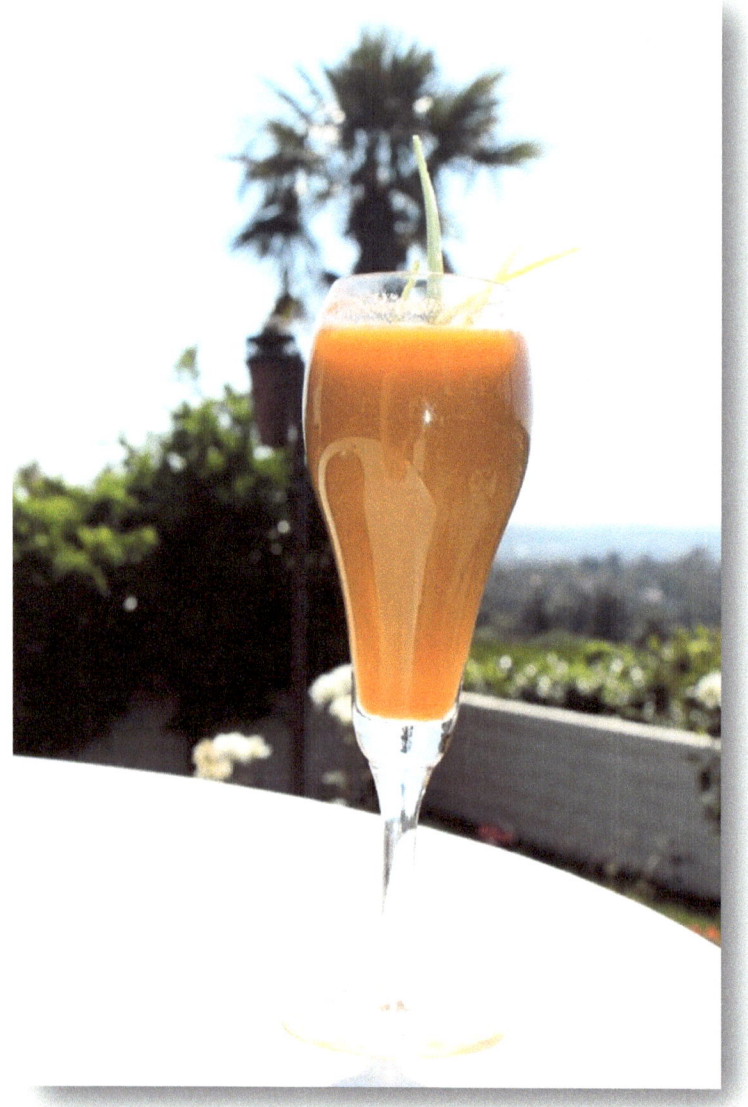

Ingredients:

- ✓ 6 Apples
- ✓ 3-4 Carrots (medium size carrots)
- ✓ ¼ tsp. Cinnamon
- ✓ ¼ tsp. nutmeg

Directions:
Juice all the ingredients, mix together and enjoy!

Evening Cleanse

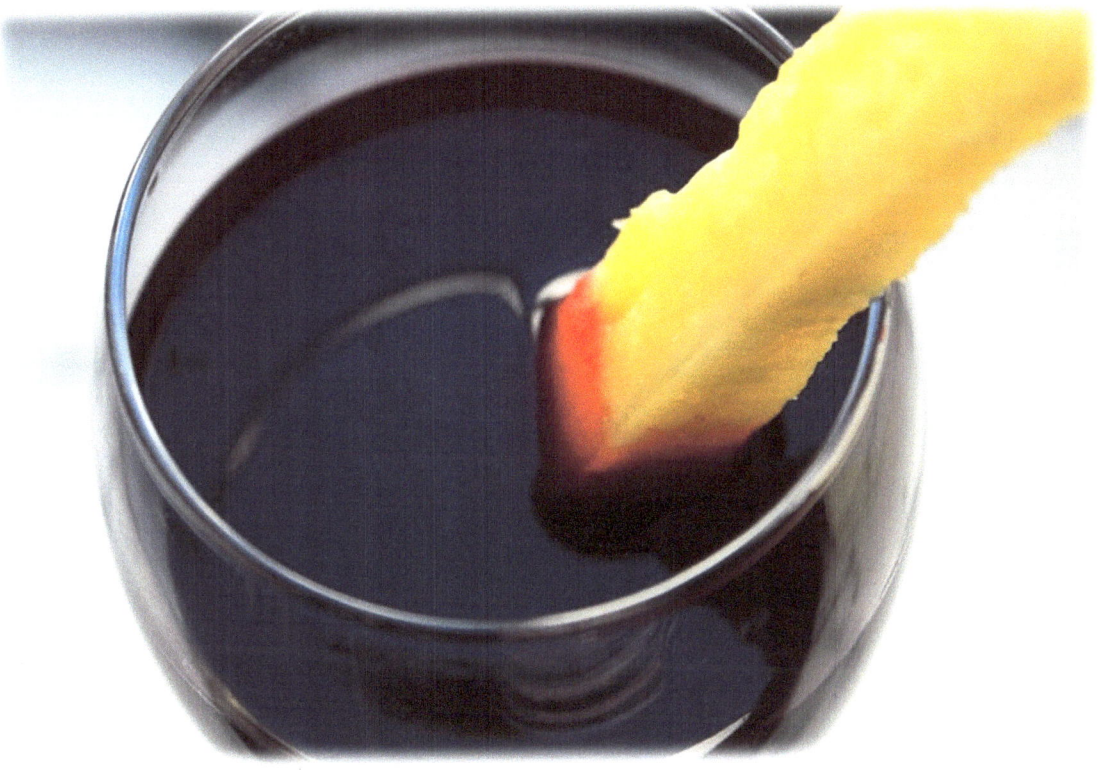

Ingredients:

- ✓ 1/3 Red Cabbage
- ✓ ½ cup Aloe Vera
- ✓ 6 Kale Leaves
- ✓ ½ Cucumber
- ✓ 1 Lime (peeled)
- ✓ 1/3 Pineapple (peeled)
- ✓ 1 Beet (peeled)
- ✓ 1 Apple

Directions:
Juice all the ingredients, mix together and enjoy!

Glow Green

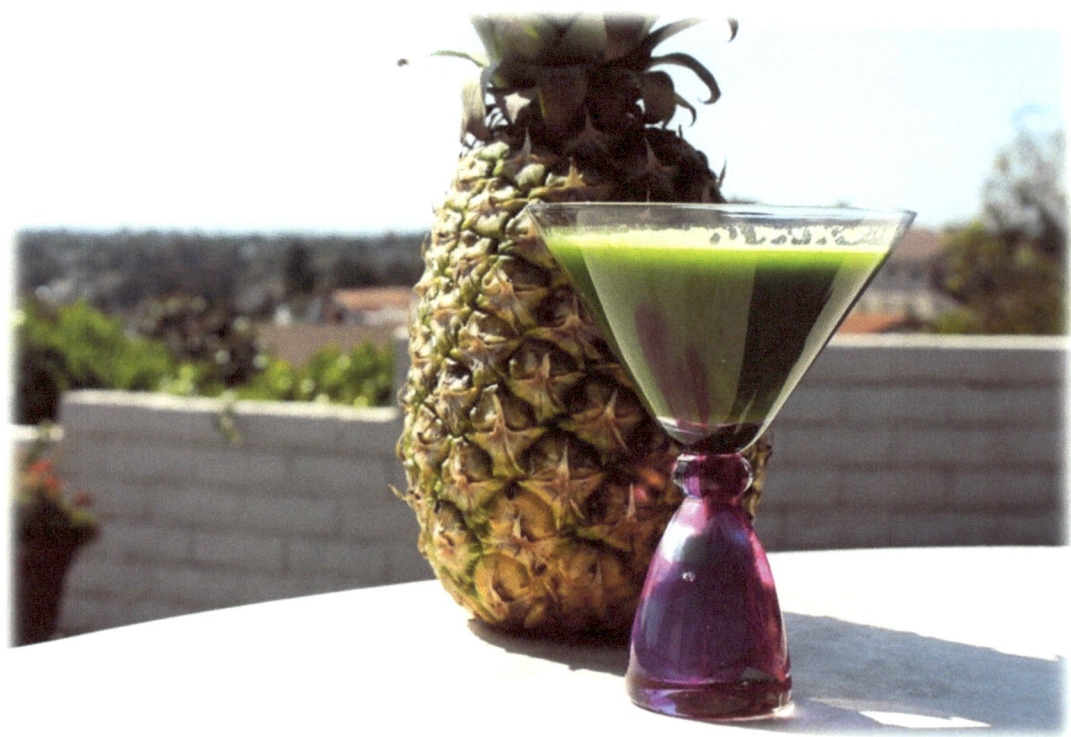

Ingredients:
- ✓ 4 Cups Spinach
- ✓ 8 Stalks of Celery
- ✓ 2 Cucumbers
- ✓ ½ bunch Parsley
- ✓ 1 Lime (peeled)
- ✓ ½ Lemon (peeled)
- ✓ ½ inch Ginger piece

Directions:
Juice all the ingredients, mix together and enjoy!

Rehydration Spark

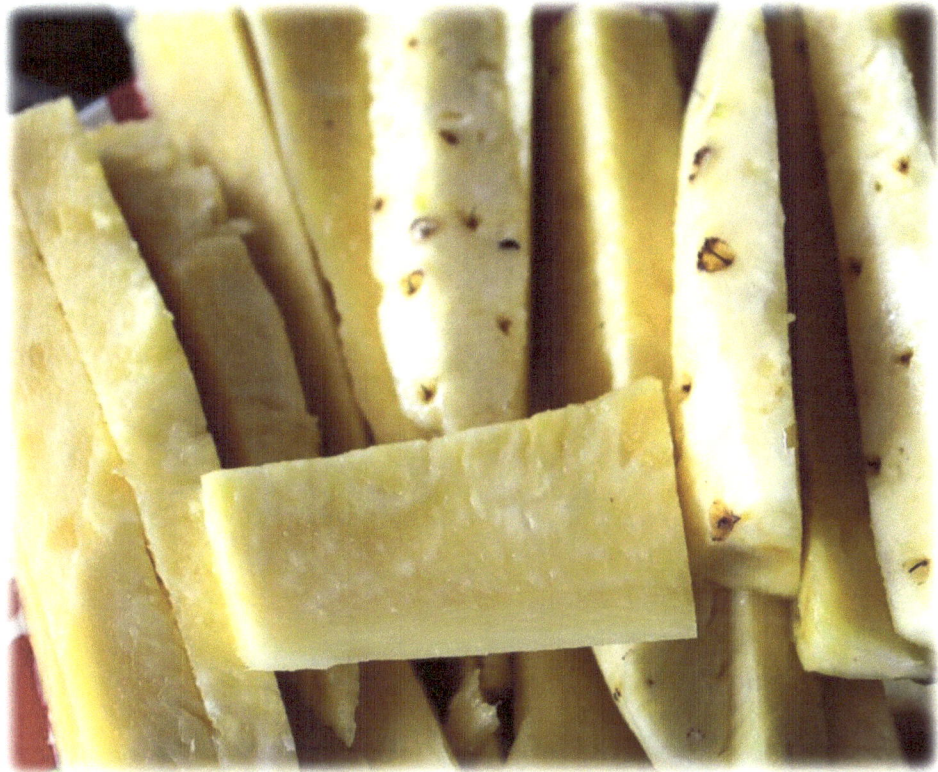

Ingredients:

- ✓ ¾ Pineapple (small pineapples)
- ✓ 6 Stalks of Celery

Directions: Juice all the ingredients, mix together and enjoy!

How to choose a good pineapple:

Choose one that is fragrant and plump with an golden color, or let it sit at room temperature until it meets the description. Slice off the bottom leaves and bottom. Then with a good knife, slice off the peel. It's not necessary to remove the center part when juicing pineapples. The center contains bromelin andIt is a great source of nutrients. Pineapple is great for the digestion of proteins!

Healthy Liver Purifier

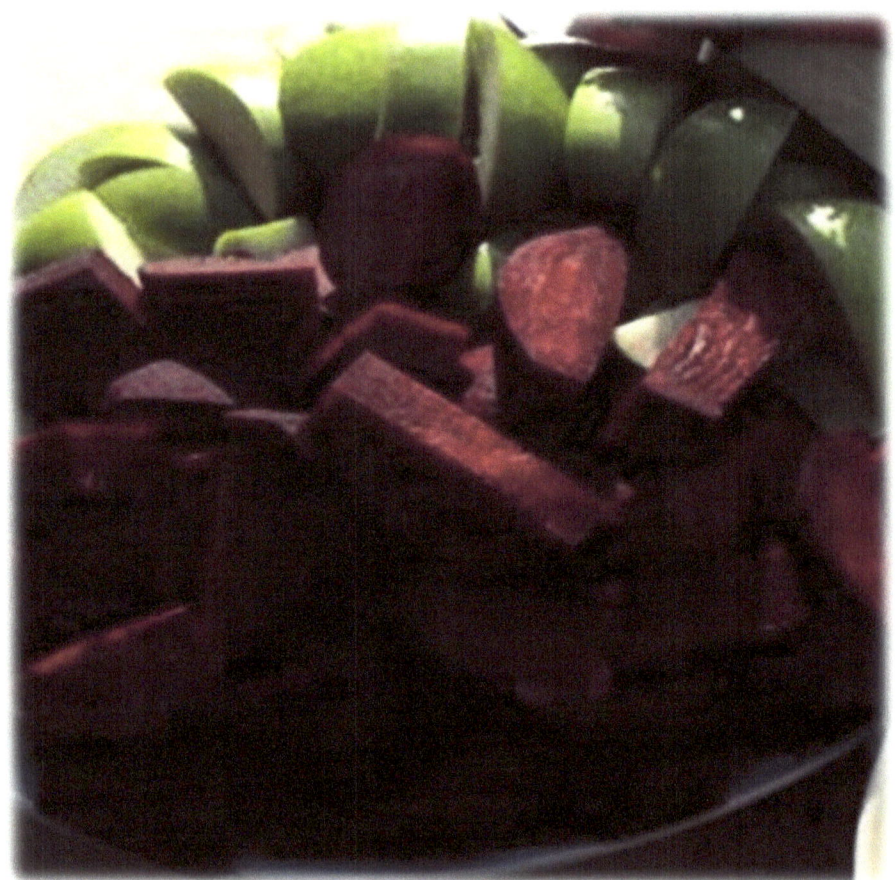

Ingredients:
- ✓ 3 medium Carrots
- ✓ 3 Celery stalks
- ✓ 3 green apples
- ✓ 2 small Beets
- ✓ 1 Cucumber
- ✓ 1 cup of parsley

Directions:
Juice all the ingredients, mix together and enjoy!

Citrus Cocktail

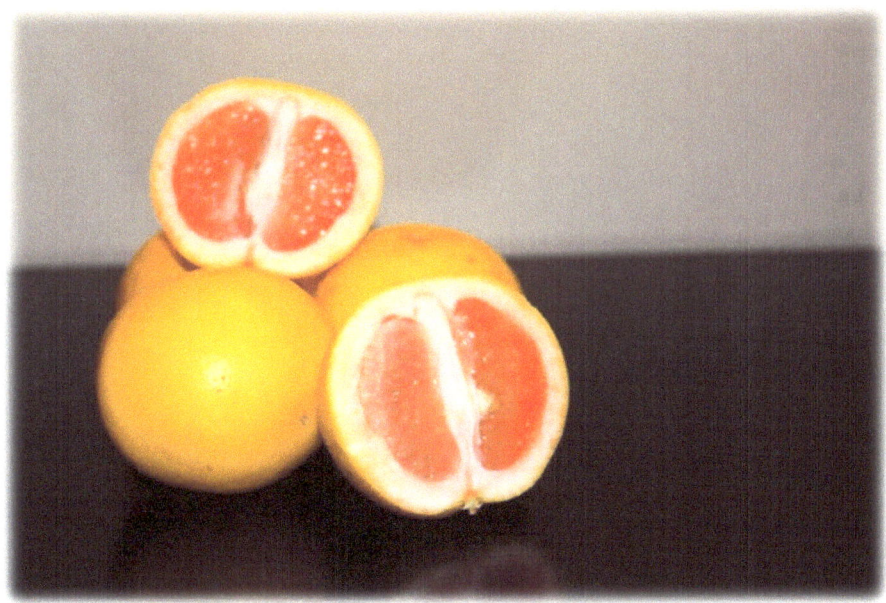

Ingredients:

- ✓ 3 Grapefruits (peeled)
- ✓ 2 oranges (peeled)
- ✓ ¼ of a pineapple (medium)
- ✓ 1 lemon (peeled)

Directions: Juice all the ingredients, mix together and enjoy!

Detox Skin Hydrator

Ingredients:

- ✓ 6 Celery stalks
- ✓ 2 cucumbers
- ✓ 1 bunch of kale
- ✓ 3 green apples

Directions: Juice all the ingredients, mix together and enjoy!

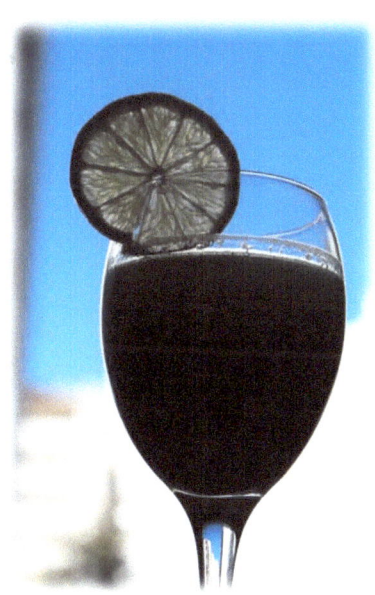

Love Chlorophyll

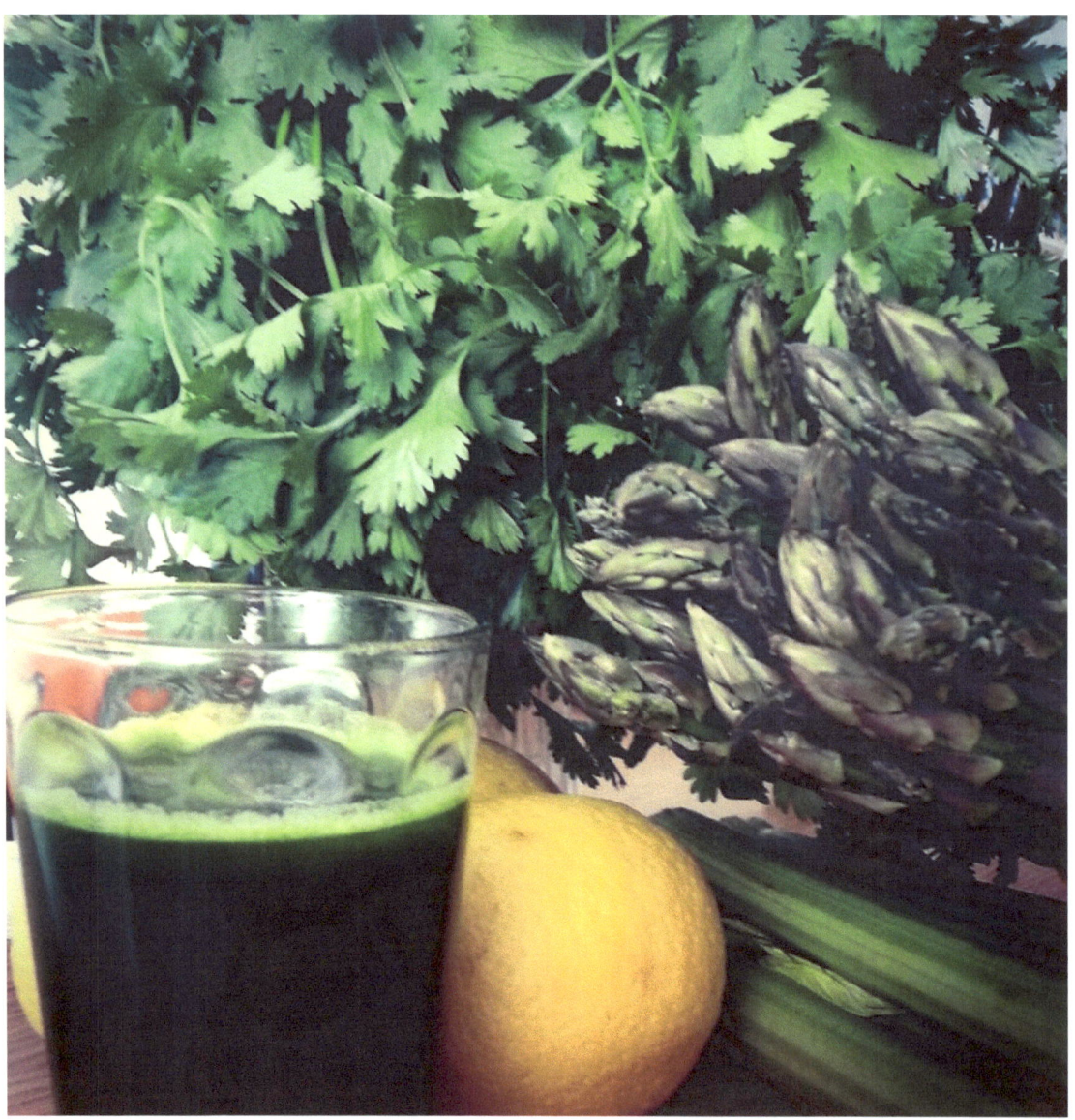

Ingredients:

- ✓ 1 oz. Wheatgrass
- ✓ 1 green apple
- ✓ 1/2 lime or lemon
- ✓ 1 inch ginger (optional)

Directions: Juice all the ingredients, mix together and enjoy!

Athlete Breakfast

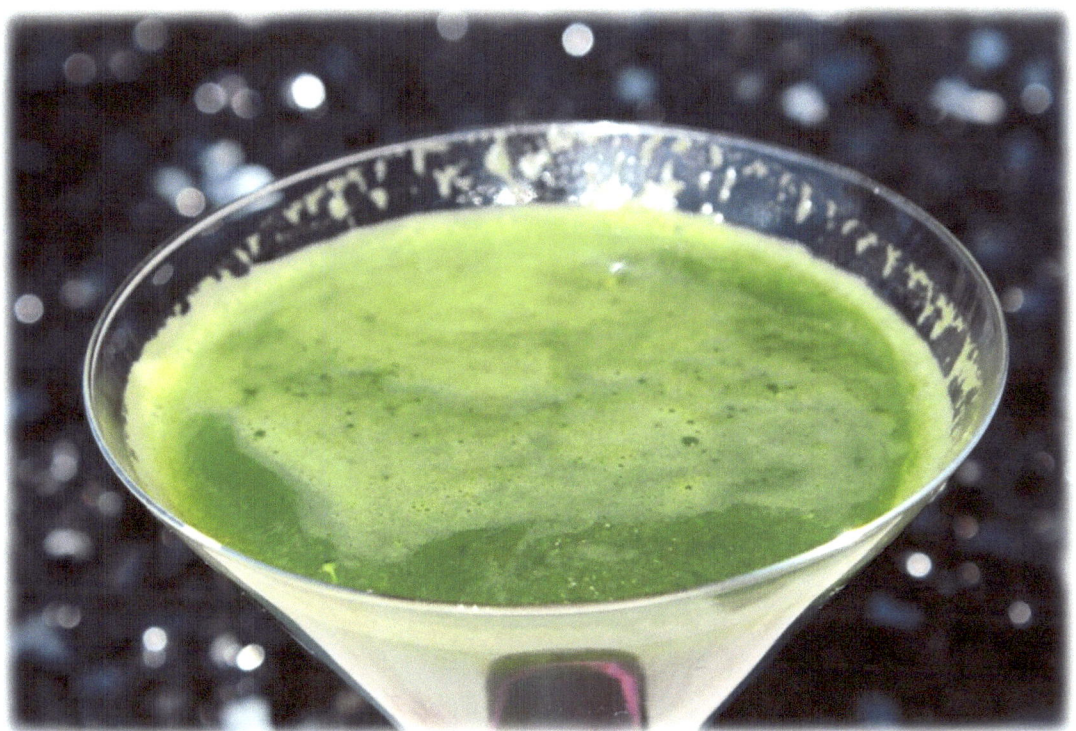

Ingredients:

- ✓ kale (4-5 leaves)
- ✓ spirulina (1 tsp)
- ✓ chlorella (1/2 tsp)
- ✓ celery (3-4 stalks)
- ✓ cucumber (1)
- ✓ lemon (1)
- ✓ cayenne (pinch)

Loaded with highly digestible protein from kale, spirulina and chlorella. Potassium from celery, cucumber for hydration, chlorophyll from all of the above, lemon to cleanse and spark digestion and cayenne for a kick.

Directions:
Juice all the ingredients, mix together and enjoy!

Green & Beet Juice

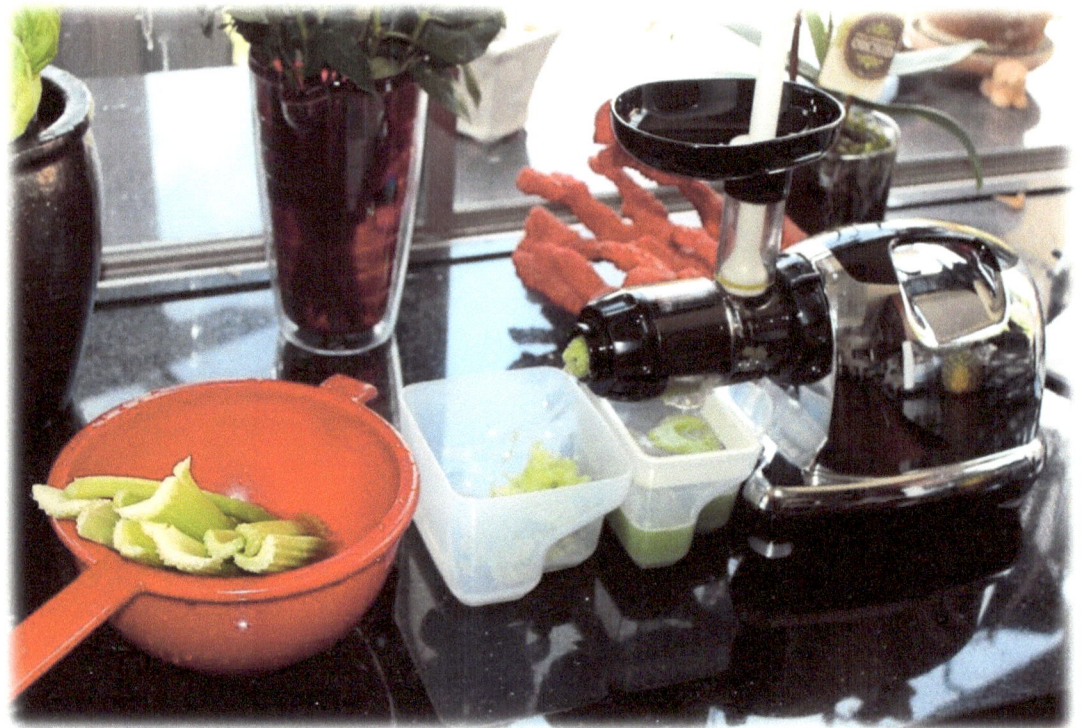

Ingredients:

- ✓ 1 Beet (small)
- ✓ 1 Cucumber
- ✓ 5 Celery Stalks
- ✓ 2 Red Apples
- ✓ 5 Leaves of Kale
- ✓ 1 Handful Spinach
- ✓ 1 Lemon (peeled)
- ✓ 3 Carrots (medium)

EXACTLY WHAT THE BODY WANTS!

Directions:
Juice all the ingredients, mix together and enjoy!

Abs Juice

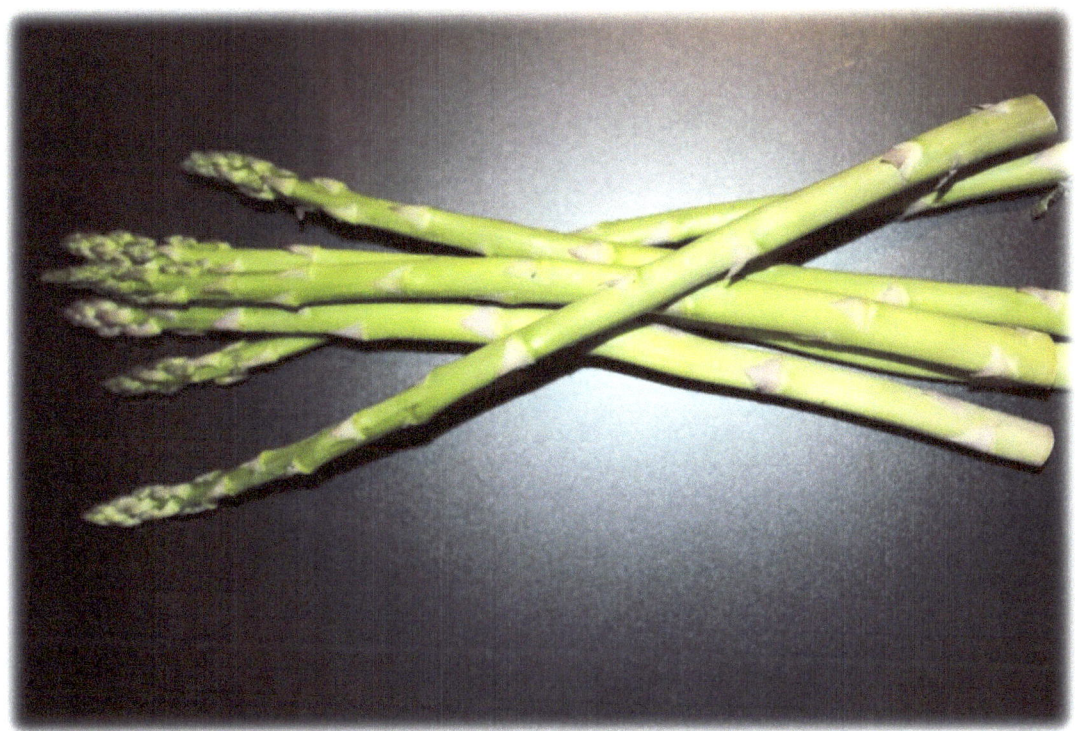

Ingredients:

- ✓ 125 g (4 oz) Asparagus spears
- ✓ 125 g (4 oz) melon
- ✓ 175 (6 oz) Cucumber
- ✓ 200 g (7 oz) pear
- ✓ 10 dandelion leaves

Directions: Juice all the ingredients, mix together and enjoy!

GOOD FOR: Bloating or water retention

This feeling can be uncomfortable and painful sometimes. It can be caused by food allergies, hormonal imbalances, a lack of essential fatty acids in the diet, and also, ironically, by not drinking enough water. Zinc is also an essential mineral to decrease water retention.

All the ingredients in the abs juice drink contain high levels of zinc and potassium. This recipe is also great if you have just eaten a salty meal.

Nutritional Information

Benefits of Each Ingredient

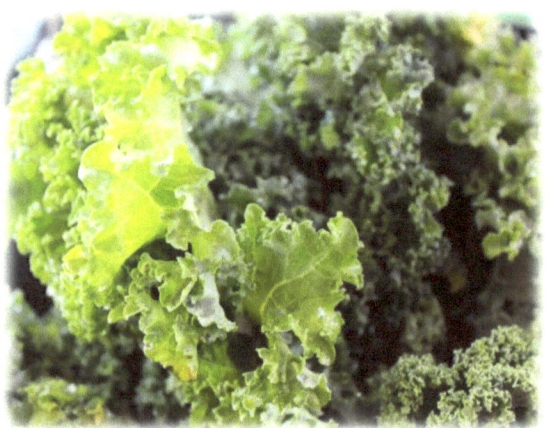 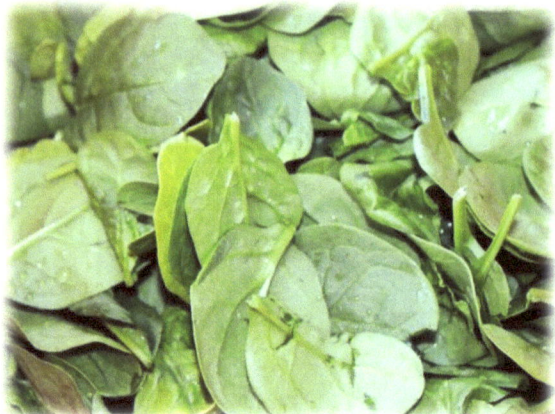

1. **Kale** – Rich in antioxidants and anti-inflammatory nutrients; Fiber and Anti-Inflammatory Omega-3 Fatty Acids; it is also high in calcium (ounce per ounce, kale has as much usable calcium as milk) is also high in chlorophyll which helps increase oxygen and nourishes and builds red blood cells.

2. **Spinach** – Rich in many nutrients, from calcium to iron, magnesium, potassium, iron, vitamin A, B-complex vitamins, calcium and magnesium. It has anti-cancer properties and strengthens immune system. Supports bone health and is also great for all kinds of health issues, from anemia to digestive problems, skin problems, etc.

3. **Romaine Lettuce** – High in silicon content, a beauty mineral which strengthens hair, nails and gives elasticity to the skin.

4. **Celery** – Neutralizes acidity because of the important minerals in this magic juice and effectively balances body's blood ph. Celery's

juice also regulates body fluid and stimulate urine production because of the minerals, potassium, and sodium, making it an important part in discarding the excess fluid in the body.

Celery is perfect for weight loss, drinking celery juice frequently throughout the day helps curb your cravings for sweets and rich foods.

5. **Cucumber** - Great for the skin and is also a mild diuretic; rich in potassium; dissolves uric acid, which causes gallstones/kidney stones; helps with digestion and regulates blood pressure.

6. **Carrots** - Strengthens the immune system and provides relief for the nervous system, alkalizing the blood and tones the walls of the intestines. It contains vitamin C, vitamin B complex, potassium, iron, sodium and phosphorus, which function to prevent illnesses and improves liver function.

   High in beta-carotene which is helpful in maintaining skin cells. Its antioxidants help prevent skin damage.

7. **Beet** – Essential nutrients are present in beet juice such as: beta-carotene, vitamin C, carotenoids, sulfur, calcium, iron, manganese and potassium choline. This drink can improve the function of the brain, cleanse blood, strengthen the gallbladder and detoxify liver. It also enhances the immune system and benefits your health in many ways.

8. **Apple** – Reduces bad cholesterol levels; helpful for weight loss; high in potassium; improves health and function of intestines. It has calcium, magnesium, phosphorus, vitamin C, beta-carotene and pectin. Apples relieves constipation, reactivates beneficial bacteria of the intestines, and helps eliminate toxins.

9. **Pineapple** – This tropical fruit is rich in vitamin C, beta-carotene, B vitamins, fiber and bromelain, the enzyme which improves digestion. Very similar to the gastric juice. It is also helpful for

weight loss.
10. Grapefruit – Excellent source of vitamin C, vitamin that helps to support the immune system; Grapefruit can also aid in reducing body fat by reducing the glycemic load of food. Lower glycemic load means less fat storage, less cravings and a better health. Just make sure not to combine medication with grapefruit because it will increase the medication's potency and can be dangerous.
11. Orange – Freshly squeezed orange juice is rich in antioxidants (vitamin C); fresh orange juices can be used to fight against some healthy issues such as heart disease and cancer; It can be used to boost your immune system and also, to reduce the harmful effects of free radicals within your body cells.
12. Lemon - Lemons clear up bad bacteria out of the system and is a natural antiseptic. It has an alkalizing effect on the body, and as it stimulates the digestive system, it purifies the liver and clear out toxins. An incredible citrus fruit.
13. Limes - Tropical fruit that belongs to the citrus group, its juice can do wonders to the body and it can relieve you from numerous diseases; Boosts the immune system and improves the body's resistance against various infections.
14. Cilantro – Strong general antioxidant properties; powerful anti-inflammatory capacities; stimulates the endocrine glands; acts as a natural ani-septic and anti-fungal agent for skin disorders like fungal infections and eczema; immune system boosting properties.
15. Ginger – Stimulates digestion; naturally freshness breath; relieves nausea; stunts the growth of cancers and tumors in the body.
16. Parsley - In herbal medicine, is used to support the urinary system. This powerful herb is a diuretic, and can help with

expelling watery poisons, excess mucus, flatulence (gas), and reducing swollen or enlarged glands. It also helps purify the blood.

17. **Jalapeno** – Reduces inflammation and since it's thermogenic, it can boost the metabolism. Jalapeno's provides potassium and some iron, and is rich in vitamins A and C.

18. **Cinnamon** - Cinnamon is a sweet and hot spice that warms and energizes the body as a whole. It supports normal function of the respiratory and digestive tracts. It helps lower blood sugar levels.

19. **Nutmeg** - Nutmeg has a sweet, nutty aroma and slightly sweet taste. It has a warming action that helps to support digestion.

20. **Cayenne Pepper** – Good for the endocrine system; increases metabolism, improves circulation, boosts the immune system and aids in digestion.

21. **Maple Syrup** – Natural Sweetener features over 54 antioxidants that can help delay or prevent diseases caused by free radicals, such as diabetes or cancer. Additionally contains high levels of manganese and zinc, keeping the heart healthy and boosting the immune system.

22. **Aloe Vera** – Aloe Vera Juice helps to detoxify the body and cleanse the colon. The properties of the juice also help to detoxify the blood stream. Improves circulation and dilates the capillaries aiding in cell growth. It also acts as an antibacterial, anti-viral and antifungal agent, preventing illness. Taking Aloe Vera juice regularly can be a feeling of energy and health.

23. **Wheatgrass** – Great source of chlorophyll. Contains alkaline properties and components to help detoxify, nourish and rebuild healthy cells. Promotes oxygen absorption into the blood stream.

24. Tomato – It contains more than 90% of water. Tomato's are antiseptic and alkaline. A raw tomato decreases liver's inflammation.

25. Broccoli – Packed with nutrients, phytonutrients and antioxidants. Provides calcium for stronger bones building.

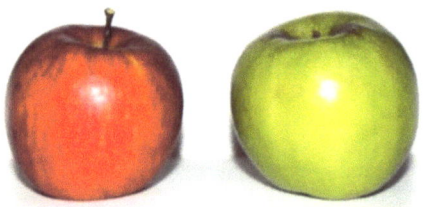

You R Ripped©

DISCLAIMER

Consult your physician before starting and following this or any nutrition plan. Each individual is different. If you have any unique or special medical needs or conditions, such as food allergies, dietary restrictions or if you are pregnant and breast feeding, please make sure you consult your medical provider before starting this nutrition plan.

www.ingramcontent.com/pod-product-compliance
Lightning Source LLC
Chambersburg PA
CBHW060817290526
45792CB00005BB/1686